STABLE MENTAL HEALTH

Contents

UNDERSTANDING MENTAL HEALTH

Mental disorders affect thinking, emotions, and behaviours. They are often associated with distress and trouble functioning in social, work, or other daily activities.

They are common. It was estimated that one in five American adults experienced mental illness in 2019 and one in 20 had a serious mental disorder.

There are many different types of mental disorders, including anxiety disorders, mood disorders, personality disorders, eating disorders, post-traumatic stress disorders, and psychotic disorders.

Many factors can contribute to the risk of mental disorders. Genetics, life experiences, and biological factors can all play a role. There is no single cause.

Effective treatment for mental disorders generally involves a combination of medications, psychotherapy, and social support and education. These treatment options can help you live well and manage your symptoms.

Anxiety Disorder

While experiencing feelings of anxiety from time to time is normal, these emotions, when they become extreme and start interfering with everyday activities can be symptoms of an anxiety disorder. The Anxiety and Depression Association of America defines anxiety disorders as specific psychiatric disorders that involve extreme fear or worry, including generalized anxiety disorder (GAD), agoraphobia, social anxiety disorder, selective mutism, separation anxiety disorder, and phobias.

Anxiety disorders are the most common mental disorders in the United States. Anxiety symptoms vary across individuals but include both psychological and physical reactions to anticipation of a threat. It is estimated that only about 40% of those suffering from an anxiety disorder receive treatment, even though the disorders are highly treatable.

Types of Anxiety Disorders

Anxiety disorders are psychiatric disorders that involve a dysregulation of the body's stress response. They differ from one another in terms of what exactly provokes the fear, anxiety, avoidance, and associated cognitive symptoms, and what type of impact they have.

Generalized Anxiety Disorder (GAD)

People with a generalized anxiety disorder (GAD) experience excessive anxiety and worry most days for at least six consecutive months. Anxious thinking can be focused on a number of circumstances, including work, relationships, and personal health.

In people with GAD, these thoughts and associated anxiety symptoms are often so persistent and overwhelming that they cause serious disruptions to everyday life and social interactions.

Other symptoms of GAD include those commonly associated with anxiety: restlessness, irritability, fatigue, and trouble sleeping.

Panic Disorder

People who have panic disorder experience repeated, unexpected panic attacks. The National Institute of Mental Health characterizes panic attacks as an abrupt surge of intense fear or discomfort that often involves a fear of disaster or of losing control even when there is no real danger. Panic attacks may result in heart racing, sweating, dizziness, and the feeling of having a heart attack.

Experiencing panic attacks can lead to a fear of panic attacks, which in turn can lead to social withdrawal and isolation. People with panic disorder may avoid places where they've previously experienced panic attacks.

Social Anxiety Disorder

Social anxiety disorder, or social phobia, is about much more than being shy. People with this anxiety disorder experience extreme fear of being judged by others and are self-conscious in social interactions to the point of avoiding them. These feelings must persist for six months to be considered to be caused by social anxiety disorder.

Separation Anxiety Disorder

People with this disorder may constantly worry about what will happen to their loved one or themselves when they are separated. Both children and adults can experience separation anxiety. When this fear of separation lasts for six or more months in adults and impairs relationships with others, it becomes a problem. Nightmares involving worst-case scenarios and physical symptoms of stress and anxiety can occur in people with this disorder.

Specific Phobias

Everyone is afraid of certain objects and situations, but when that fear turns into feelings of intense anxiety or dread that lasts six or more months, and interferes with your life, it may indicate a phobia. Specific phobia is an intense, irrational fear of something that poses little or no actual danger. While the specific source of fear can differ from person to person, phobias are a type of anxiety disorder that can severely impair someone's ability to function in everyday situations. Phobias can be of spiders (arachnophobia), the dark (nyctophobia), clowns (coulrophobia), repetitive patterns of holes (trypophobia), and many others.

Agoraphobia

People with agoraphobia have a disabling fear of any places or situations where escape seems challenging if they panic or feel embarrassed. This fear goes beyond what may be rational and influences behavior. It involves avoidance of situations such as being alone outside of the home, traveling in a car, bus, or airplane, or being in a crowded area.

What Is Selective Mutism?

Selective mutism is a somewhat rare disorder commonly associated with anxiety. It results in a failure to speak in specific social situations despite having normal language skills. This disorder usually presents before the age of 5. Other associated behaviors may include extreme shyness, fear of social embarrassment, compulsive traits, withdrawal, clinging behavior, and temper tantrums.

How Do I Know If I Have an Anxiety Disorder?

Everybody experiences anxiety, but only some will develop an anxiety disorder that requires diagnosis, treatment, and follow-up.

Symptoms

While each specific disorder comes with its own anxiety symptoms, there are tell-tale signs that anxiety is becoming unmanageable or is beginning to disrupt daily functioning.

Symptoms common to all anxiety disorders include:

- Difficulty sleeping
- Dizziness
- Dry mouth
- Feelings of nervousness, panic, fear, and unease
- Muscle tightness
- Nausea

- Rapid or irregular heartbeat
- Sweaty or cold hands and/or feet
- Tingling or numbness in the hands or feet
- Unable to be calm or hold still

If you notice these symptoms and they last six months or longer, you may have an anxiety disorder.

Diagnosis

Getting a diagnosis can be the first step to getting treatment. While there is no definitive test for anxiety, if symptoms are present and persistent, your healthcare provider may conduct a physical assessment and may run diagnostic tests to rule out potential medical causes.6

If no physical illness is found to be causing your symptoms, you will be referred to a psychiatrist or another mental health professional to be evaluated for an anxiety disorder. They will use the standard reference manual for diagnosing recognized mental illnesses in the United States, the Diagnostic and Statistical Manual of Mental Disorders 5th Edition (DSM-5), to determine if you have an anxiety disorder. The diagnostic criteria for each anxiety disorder are different.

You may be asked questions like whether you worry more days than not and if you've noticed any physical symptoms such as restlessness, feeling tired easily, trouble concentrating, irritability, muscle tension, or trouble sleeping.

Risk Factors

Anxiety disorders are influenced by both genetic and environmental factors. While risk factors for each anxiety disorder vary, some factors associated with developing an anxiety disorder are common across different types:

- Adverse childhood experiences, including neglect or abuse

- Temperamental traits of shyness or behavioral inhibition in childhood
- A history of anxiety or other mental illnesses in the family

Some physical health conditions, such as thyroid problems or heart arrhythmias, are also commonly associated with anxiety. For example, there is a high prevalence of psychiatric symptoms and disorders in thyroid disease. Heart arrhythmias or palpitations are also associated with anxiety and can be induced by stress.

Caffeine or other stimulants and some medications can also trigger or aggravate symptoms of anxiety disorders.

How Can I Get Help if I Have Severe Anxiety?

Severe anxiety requires treatment. Your mental health professional may decide that one or two of the following options or a combination of all three is ideal for treating and managing your anxiety disorder.

Psychotherapy

Cognitive behavioral therapy, or CBT, is a short-term form of psychotherapy that has been proven to be an effective form of treatment for anxiety disorders. If avoidance of feared situations is a relevant factor in phobic disorders, exposure techniques should be included in the treatment schedule, in which patients are confronted with their feared situations. It has been shown that only a few sessions (e.g., one to five) may be necessary for effective treatment of specific phobias.

Medication

Pharmacological therapies are commonly prescribed to alleviate the symptoms of anxiety disorders, including anti-anxiety medications. The most common one used for anxiety disorders is benzodiazepine, which are effective in relieving anxiety and take effect quickly, but people can build up a resistance to it. Buspirone is a non-benzodiazepine medication specifically used to treat chronic anxiety, although it does not help everyone.

Antidepressants like selective serotonin reuptake inhibitors and serotonin-norepinephrine reuptake inhibitors are also prescribed to treat anxiety disorders. People with anxiety disorders can also be treated with other medications such as pregabalin, tricyclic antidepressants, moclobemide, and more.

Be mindful of the following when taking medications to manage anxiety disorder symptoms:

• Keep your provider informed about your symptoms. If a medicine isn't controlling symptoms, its dosage may need to be changed or you may need to try a new medicine.

- Do not change the dosage or stop taking the medicine without talking to your provider.
- Take medicine at set times. For example, take it every day at breakfast. Check with your provider about the best time to take your medicine.
- Ask your provider about side effects and what to do if they occur.

Antidepressants have been associated with increased risk of suicidality (suicidal thinking and behavior) in children and adolescents.

Self-Care

Self-care is an essential part of mental health care. The World Health Organization defines self-care as a broad concept that also encompasses hygiene (general and personal); nutrition (type and quality of food eaten); lifestyle (sporting activities, leisure, etc.); environmental factors (living conditions, social habits, etc.); socioeconomic factors (income level, cultural beliefs, etc.); and self-medication.

Some self-care tips for people with anxiety disorders include:

- Getting enough sleep
- Eating healthy foods

- Keeping a regular daily schedule
- Getting out of the house every day
- Exercising every day. Even a little bit of exercise, such as a 15-minute walk, can help
- Stay away from alcohol and street drugs
- Talk with family or friends when feeling nervous or frightened
- Find out about different types of group activities available

Life is filled with different stressors, and we all experience some form of anxiety every day. When anxiety levels are high for a long period of time, however, you may have an anxiety disorder. These disorders can be persistent and disabling, but fortunately, there are several effective treatment options.

Besides therapy and medications, you can also be proactive about managing your symptoms by taking good care of yourself. Maintaining a positive mindset and keeping yourself healthy will go a long way toward minimizing disruptions from your anxiety and improving your quality of life.

What Are Affective (Mood) Disorders?

Affective disorders, also known as mood disorders, are mental disorders that primarily affect a person's emotional state. They impact the way they think, feel, and go about daily life.

There are many types of mood disorders, including major depressive disorder and bipolar disorder, among others.

Symptoms vary by condition and from person to person. It is estimated that 21.4% of adults in the United States will experience some type of mood disorder throughout their lives.

Mood disorders are not the same as normal mood fluctuations. Fluctuations in mood are a normal response to everyday occurrences and stressors, and usually do not negatively affect one's quality of life and overall ability to function.

Mood disorders, on the other hand, can greatly affect one's quality of life, causing issues with one's relationships, career, and self-esteem.

Those who struggle with mood disorders may find relief through therapy, medications, and lifestyle changes.

Symptoms

Symptoms vary in intensity and by disorder. Two of the most common mood disorders are depression, or major depressive disorder (MDD), and bipolar disorder.

Depression

There are several different types of depression, including:

- Major depression: Having less interest in usual activities, experiencing a depressed mood such as feeling sad or hopeless, and other symptoms for at least two weeks
- Dysthymia (also known as persistent depressive disorder): Having chronic depressed moods accompanied by other symptoms for at least two years

Depression can have several specifiers that further characterize the mood disorder, including:

- Seasonal affective disorder (SAD): Having depressive symptoms that recur at certain times of the year, usually during the winter months
- Psychotic depression, or major depressive disorder with psychotic features: Experiencing severe depression plus some form of psychosis, such as having disturbing false fixed beliefs (delusions) or hearing or seeing upsetting things that others cannot hear or see (hallucinations)
- Depression with peripartum onset or postpartum depression: Experiencing a depressive episode during pregnancy or shortly after giving birth

Symptoms of depression can include:

- Excessive and sometimes unexplained sadness
- Hopelessness
- Loss of interest in favorite activities
- Appetite and weight changes
- Feelings of guilt
- Low self-esteem
- Memory issues
- Oversleeping or insomnia
- Agitation
- Suicidal ideation or attempts

Bipolar Disorder

Bipolar disorders are generally marked by shifts between depressive (extremely low mood) and manic (extremely elevated or irritable mood) episodes. There are several types of bipolar disorder. They include:

- Bipolar I: The most severe form, with periods of full-blown mania
- Bipolar II: Experiencing episodes of depression alternating with periods of hypomania, a form of mania that's less severe
- Cyclothymia: Alternating between symptoms of hypomania and depression for more than two years

- Unspecified bipolar disorder: When symptoms are characteristic of bipolar disorder but do not meet the diagnostic criteria of the any of the other types of bipolar disorders

During mania, one may experience:

- Increased energy
- Racing thoughts
- Decreased ability and need for sleep
- Flight of ideas
- Grandiose thoughts
- Reckless behavior

During a depressive episode as a part of a bipolar illness, one may experience symptoms similar to those of major depressive disorder, including sadness, low self-esteem, cognitive issues, and suicidal ideation.

Premenstrual Dysmorphic Disorder (PMDD)

Premenstrual dysmorphic disorder (PMDD) is a type of depressive disorder that is a severe form of premenstrual syndrome (PMS). It involves a combination of symptoms that people can experience about a week or two before their period.

Symptoms of PMDD include:

- Severe mood swings
- Anger and irritability

- Increased appetite
- Depression
- Insomnia or sleeping more
- Feeling a loss of control

Causes

Mood disorders can be caused by a combination of factors, including chemical imbalances in the brain, genetics, and stressful life events.

Chemical Imbalances

Neurons are the building blocks of the brain and nervous system. Neurons communicate with other neurons, glands, and muscles through the release of substances known as neurotransmitters. These chemicals are involved in everything, from our basic biological functions, such as breathing, to our fight-or-flight response.

Neurotransmitters are also involved in the regulation of moods and emotions. A number of neurotransmitters are involved in mood disorders. One that plays an integral role in the development or susceptibility to depression is serotonin. Lower levels of serotonin may contribute to depression.

Other neurotransmitters commonly associated with mood disorders include dopamine and norepinephrine.

Brain Structure

Brain structure is also believed to play a role in depression. Researchers have found one area in the brain, the hippocampus, is smaller in depressed patients. They believe the reason for this may be because extended, ongoing exposure to stress hormones hindered the growth of nerve cells within that brain region.

Other brain structures potentially involved in mood disorders include the amygdala and thalamus.

Genetics

Genetics are a significant factor involved in the susceptibility of mood disorders, and mood disorders are known to run in families.

Life Events and Changes

Stressful life events and changes, including starting a new job, moving, and other transitional periods, can also spark a mood disorder such as depression.

Diagnosis

There is not a single test for determining if one has a mood disorder. Rather, a healthcare provider will conduct a psychiatric evaluation and take note of all the symptoms someone is experiencing to determine the correct diagnosis.

Healthcare providers use the Diagnostic and Statistical Manual of Mental Disorders, 5th Edition (DSM-5) to diagnose mental disorders, including mood disorders.8 This guide contains diagnostic criteria for each mental disorder.

Depression

In order to be diagnosed with depression, you must experience symptoms for at least two weeks. However, this timeline will differ based on the specific type of depression you are experiencing. For example:

• Dysthymia: Symptoms must be present for two years or more.

• Major depressive disorder with a peripartum onset: Symptoms must be present during pregnancy or within four weeks of giving birth.

- Seasonal affective disorder (SAD): Symptoms must be recurrent during a particular time of year, usually the winter months.

Depression appears differently in every person, and no two cases are the same. As such, not every symptom will be experienced by each person diagnosed with depression. However, several persistent symptoms must be present within the timeframe specified for the given depression type to qualify.

Bipolar Disorder

Healthcare providers diagnose bipolar disorder based on symptoms, experiences, and histories.

One must experience at least one episode of mania or hypomania to be diagnosed with bipolar I disorder, as well as a depressive episode that lasts at least two weeks to be diagnosed with bipolar II disorder.

Treatment

Options for treating affective disorders include medications and therapy. Lifestyle changes, such as increasing exercise, eating a healthy diet, and reducing stress, may also help. Because of the complexity of factors involved in mood disorders, it is vital to approach treatment from different angles.

Usually, a combination of medication and therapy is recommended. Keep in mind, however, that treatment plans will vary based on individual needs. It's best to talk to your healthcare provider for your own best course of action.

Medications

Various psychiatric medications are available for the treatment of various mood disorders. Each of these interacts with neurotransmitter levels in the brain to help treat any potential imbalances.

Some common medications prescribed to help treat mood disorders include:

- Selective serotonin reuptake inhibitors (SSRIs)

- Serotonin–norepinephrine reuptake inhibitors (SNRIs)
- Antipsychotics
- Mood stabilizers

Therapy

Psychotherapy is another option for treatment. However, therapy is not one-size-fits-all and there are many options.

Common therapies used for the treatment of mood disorders include:

- Cognitive behavioral therapy (CBT): CBT focuses on reworking negative, disruptive thought patterns. It is used in treating both depression and bipolar disorder.

- Dialectical behavioral therapy (DBT): DBT was originally created for the treatment of borderline personality disorder (BPD), but has since shown to be helpful in managing moods in cases of depression and bipolar disorder as well.

Lifestyle

Lifestyle can contribute to better management of mood disorders. Some changes that can help include:

- Engage in regular exercise: Exercise can be beneficial in the treatment of mood disorders.
- Build healthy relationships: The people you surround yourself with have a huge impact on your well-being. Maintaining strong,

healthy, and nourishing relationships with your loved ones can vastly improve your mental health.

- Focus on sleep: Practicing proper sleep hygiene is imperative to managing depression. There are a number of known best practices for getting better sleep.

- Avoid alcohol: Excessive and persistent drinking increases your odds of developing depression. Drinking in moderation or avoiding it is recommended for those who struggle with a mood disorder.

Coping

Living with a mood disorder is no easy feat. Affective disorders can touch every area of life, from relationships to careers to self-esteem to physical health. However, it is possible to live well despite the difficulties that come with these types of mental disorders.

Focusing on sleep hygiene, getting support from friends and family, getting regular exercise, eating healthy, and staying away from substances can vastly improve your quality of life if you are living with a mood disorder.

Joining a support group can help you feel less alone in your struggles as well. Organizations that can be helpful in finding support include the National Alliance on Mental Illness

(NAMI) and Substance Abuse and Mental Health Services Administration.

What Is Clinical Depression?

Clinical depression, also called major depression or major depressive disorder (MDD), is often confused with having a sad or low mood. Although feeling sad is one symptom of clinical depression, there must be several other signs and symptoms—in addition to sadness—for someone to be formally diagnosed with clinical depression.

Clinical depression is considered a potentially chronic and severe disorder with medical comorbidities and high mortality.

Understanding the signs and symptoms of clinical depression are important to ensure someone can receive an accurate diagnosis and treatment.

What Is Clinical Depression?

Clinical depression is a serious form of mental illness that impacts more than just a person's mood. It affects the way a person:2

- Thinks
- Acts
- Feels
- Manages their life

A diagnosis of clinical depression means that a person has symptoms that interfere with the ability to function at work and home, which adversely impacts the way a person is able to enjoy hobbies and leisure activities, socialization, relationships, and more.

Clinical depression involves more than just emotions, it encompasses physical symptoms—such as inability to sleep and loss of appetite—as well. It's important to note that clinical depression is a set of signs and symptoms that may reflect a chemical imbalance in the brain.

Symptoms

Some of the most pervasive symptoms of clinical depression are a severe and persistent low mood, profound sadness, or a sense of despair. The characteristics, symptoms, or traits of depression may vary in severity from very mild to severe. Symptoms may include:

- An ongoing feeling of sadness or depressed mood
- Loss of interest in hobbies and activities that are usually enjoyable
- Low energy level or a feeling of fatigue
- Insomnia (trouble sleeping) or sleeping too much
- Loss of appetite and subsequent weight loss
- Eating too much, resulting in weight gain

- Slowed movement or speech
- Increase in activity (pacing, nervous gestures such as wringing hands repeatedly)
- Feelings of guilt or worthlessness
- Trouble concentrating
- Difficulty making decisions
- Thoughts of suicide (or an active plan to commit suicide)
- Obsession with death

For a formal diagnosis of clinical depression, these symptoms must last at least two weeks and they must represent a change from the former level of functioning experienced before symptoms began and they must cause a person significant impairment or distress in their job, social situations, or other areas of functioning. The symptoms must not be caused by another medical condition, including substance abuse.

Other physical conditions that can mimic the symptoms of depression include:

- Thyroid problems
- A brain tumor
- A vitamin deficiency

Diagnosis

A diagnosis of clinical depression often begins with a physical examination, lab tests, and other diagnostic measures to rule out any physical conditions such as thyroid problems. After which, the primary healthcare provider may refer you to a psychiatrist or other mental health professional (such as a psychologist licensed clinical social worker or LICSW) for an evaluation. An evaluation by a mental health professional may include:

- A psychiatric evaluation: This includes a history of current symptoms and an assessment of your thoughts, feelings, and behaviors. You may be asked to answer some questions in written form.

- A family history: This is used to decipher whether there is any mental illness in your family.

• A diagnostic evaluation: This evaluates your symptoms as compared to the DSM-5, a diagnostic tool called the Diagnostic and Statistical Manual of Mental Disorders.

Causes

The exact cause of clinical depression is unknown, anyone can suffer from major depressive disorder. However, there are some known causes linked with clinical depression, these include:

• Biochemistry: Specific brain chemicals are thought to play a role in symptoms of depression.

• Genetics: Depression is known to run in families. If you have a parent or sibling with clinical depression, you have a two to three times higher likeliness of developing depression, compared to someone who does not have this family link.6

- Environmental factors: Such as being exposed to violence, or abuse and neglect, particularly during childhood, can increase a person's likeliness of depression.5 Poverty is also known to make a person more vulnerable to clinical depression.

Risk Factors

While no one can predict exactly if a person will become depressed, there are some risk factors that increase the likeliness of being diagnosed with depression, these include:7

- Having had a previous clinical depression episode
- Having a family history of depression, alcoholism, bipolar disorder, or a family member who has committed suicide
- Having substance abuse problems
- Going through significant life changes (such as the loss of a loved one)
- Having high levels of stress
- Having experienced a trauma
- Having certain medical conditions (such as a brain tumor)
- Taking some types of medications known to cause depression

- Having certain personality characteristics (such as being extremely pessimistic or having low self-esteem)

Types

There are several different types of depression that a person can have; the primary difference is the features involved. You may or may not have what is called a specifier linked with depression, these specifiers may include:

- Anxious distress: Depression, along with feelings of restlessness, being worried, keyed up, or tense.

- Mixed features: Depression, along with increased energy, excessive talking, inflated sense of self-esteem (also referred to as mania or manic).

- Melancholic features: Severe depression, linked with early rising, loss of all interest in things that you previously enjoyed, worsened mood in the morning, and guilty feelings.
- Atypical features: Depression with features that include a mood that can brighten in response to positive events, an increase in appetite, excessive sleep, a heavy feeling in the arms or legs (called leaden paralysis).
- Psychotic features: Depression accompanied by psychosis, such as hallucinations or delusions.

- Peripartum onset: Occurs during pregnancy or within four weeks of giving birth.
- Seasonal Pattern: Also known as seasonal affective disorder, involves depression that is linked with a specific season of the year (usually with lower sunlight exposure, such as fall or winter). Symptoms may include trouble getting up and going to work during the winter months.

Treatment

Clinical depression is one of the most treatable of all mental health disorders.2 In fact, between 80 to 90% of people with depression respond favorably to treatment.2

Medication

When the chemistry in the brain is contributing to a person's depression, your healthcare provider may prescribe an antidepressant. Antidepressants are not considered habit-forming drugs, they simply help to modify the brain chemistry, thus improving symptoms of depression.

One drawback of antidepressants is that they can take up to several weeks to begin having a therapeutic effect (lowering symptoms of depression).

If you start taking antidepressants and do not see any improvement in your symptoms after several weeks, your psychiatrist may adjust your dose, or add an additional medication.

Usually, you will be instructed by your healthcare provider to take your antidepressants for at least six months (or longer) after you see improvement in symptoms; you may be advised to take the medication long-term, to reduce the risk of future episodes of depression.

Psychotherapy

Psychotherapy—sometimes referred to as "talk therapy"—is a common treatment for mild depression. If you have moderate to severe depression, you may be encouraged to engage in talk therapy, along with antidepressant medications.

A variety of psychotherapy modalities have been found helpful for depression. One of the most effective modes of talk therapy for depression is called cognitive behavioral therapy (CBT), a type of psychological treatment that has been found to be effective for many different issues, such as:

- Depression
- Anxiety
- Alcohol and substance use disorders
- Eating disorders
- Other types of mental illness

CBT therapy involves various strategies; some or all of these strategies may be employed during individual or group therapy, they include:

• Learning to recognize distortions in thinking that lead to problems and reevaluate these distortions

• Learning to change behavioral patterns (such as facing fears when a person suffers from severe anxiety)

• Learning problem-solving skills and how to employ them in specific situations

• Learning how to gain confidence in one's strengths and abilities

- Adopting improved insight into the motivation and behavior of others
- Learning how to calm the mind and relax the body

The time it takes for the treatment of depression can vary, depending on several factors including:

- The severity of clinical depression
- The extent of trauma one may have experienced
- Whether a person has co-occurring conditions, such as substance use disorder
- The type of depression a person has

ECT Therapy

Electroconvulsive therapy (ECT) is a treatment for depression that is very effective, but is usually reserved for those who do not respond well to other types of treatment, such as medication. ECT is much different today than historically, when a person was awake during the process. This treatment modality began during the 1940s. Today, however, ECT is done under anesthesia. It involves a very brief electrical stimulation to the brain after the person has been put to sleep. ECT is usually comprised of approximately six to 12 sessions.

Coping

There are many things you can do to help you cope with clinical depression, some of the most common interventions include lifestyle changes such as:

- Ensuring that you get enough sleep each night
- Eating a healthy diet
- Getting involved in a daily physical workout routine (with the okay from your healthcare provider). Studies have shown exercise can mitigate depression.
- Avoiding the use of alcohol (which is a depressant) and other drugs

- Adopting measures to manage stress (such as deep breathing and relaxation techniques, yoga, or mindfulness practice.

MENTAL HEALTH AND EXERCISE

There are many reasons why physical activity is good for your body – having a healthy heart and improving your joints and bones are just two, but did you know that physical activity is also beneficial for your mental health and wellbeing?

What is physical activity?

At a very basic level, physical activity means any movement of your body that uses your muscles and expends energy. One of the great things about physical activity is that there are endless possibilities and there will be an activity to suit almost everyone!

It is recommended that the average adult should do between 75 and 150 minutes of exercise a week. This can be either moderate intensity exercise, such as walking, hiking or riding a bike, or it can be more vigorous activities, such as running, swimming fast, aerobics or skipping with a rope. Any activity that raises your heart rate, makes you breathe faster, and makes you feel warmer counts towards your exercise!

An easy way to look at types of physical activity is to put them into four separate categories.

Daily physical activity

For adults, physical activity can include recreational or leisure-time physical activity,

transportation (e.g. walking or cycling), occupational activity (i.e. work), household chores, play, games, sports, or planned exercise in the context of daily, family, and community activities.

Everyday things such as walking to the bus stop, carrying bags or climbing stairs all count, and can add up to the 150 minutes of exercise a week recommended for the average adult.

Exercise

Purposeful activity carried out to improve health or fitness, such as jogging or cycling, or lifting weights to increase strength.

Play

Unstructured activity that is done for fun or enjoyment.

Sport

Structured and competitive activities that include anything from football or squash to cricket. We can play these as part of a team or even on our own. This can be a fun and interactive way of getting exercise that doesn't have to feel like exercising.

These activities can vary in intensity and can include high-intensity activities, such as tennis, athletics, swimming, and keep-fit classes, or they can be lower-intensity activities and sports, such as snooker or darts. Making exercise fun rather than something you have to do can be a motivator to keep it up.

What is wellbeing?

The government defines wellbeing as 'a positive physical, social and mental state'. For our purposes, we are focusing on mental wellbeing.

Mental wellbeing does not have a single universal definition, but it does encompass factors such as:

☐ The sense of feeling good about ourselves and being able to function well individually or in relationships

☐ The ability to deal with the ups and downs of life, such as coping with challenges and making the most of opportunities

☐ The feeling of connection to our community and surroundings

☐ Having control and freedom over our lives

☐ Having a sense of purpose and feeling valued

Of course, mental wellbeing does not mean being happy all the time, and it does not mean that you won't experience negative or painful emotions, such as grief, loss, or failure, which are a part of normal life. However, whatever your age, being physically active can help you to lead a mentally healthier life and can improve your wellbeing.

What impact does physical activity have on wellbeing?

Physical activity has a huge potential to enhance our wellbeing. Even a short burst of 10 minutes' brisk walking increases our mental alertness, energy and positive mood.

Participation in regular physical activity can increase our self-esteem and can reduce stress and anxiety. It also plays a role in preventing the development of mental health problems and in improving the quality of life of people experiencing mental health problems.

Impact on our mood

Physical activity has been shown to have a positive impact on our mood. A study asked people to rate their mood immediately after periods of physical activity (e.g. going for a walk or doing housework), and periods of inactivity (e.g. reading a book or watching television). Researchers found that the participants felt more content, more awake and calmer after being physically active compared to after periods of inactivity. They also found that the effect of physical activity on mood was greatest when mood was initially low.

There are many studies looking at physical activity at different levels of intensity and its impact on people's mood. Overall, research has found that low-intensity aerobic exercise – for 30–35 minutes, 3–5 days a week, for 10–12 weeks – was best at increasing positive moods (e.g. enthusiasm, alertness).

Impact on our stress

When events occur that make us feel threatened or that upset our balance in some way, our body's defences cut in and create a stress response, which may make us feel a variety of uncomfortable physical symptoms and make us behave differently, and we may also experience emotions more intensely.

The most common physical signs of stress include sleeping problems, sweating, and loss of appetite. Symptoms like these are triggered by a rush of stress hormones in our body – otherwise known as the 'fight or flight' response. It is these hormones, adrenaline and noradrenaline, which raise our blood pressure, increase our heart rate and increase the rate at which we perspire, preparing our body for an emergency response. They can also reduce blood flow to our skin and can reduce our stomach activity, while cortisol, another stress hormone, releases fat and sugar into the system to boost our energy.

Physical exercise can be very effective in relieving stress. Research on employed adults has found that highly active individuals tend to have lower stress rates compared to individuals who are less active.

Impact on our self-esteem

Exercise not only has a positive impact on our physical health, but it can also increase our self-esteem. Self-esteem is how we feel about ourselves and how we perceive our self-worth. It is a key indicator of our mental wellbeing and our ability to cope with life stressors.

Physical activity has been shown to have a positive influence on our self-esteem and self-worth. This relationship has been found in children, adolescents, young adults, adults and older people, and across both males and females.

Dementia and cognitive decline in older people

Improvements in healthcare have led to an increasing life expectancy and a growing population of people over 65 years. Alongside this increase in life expectancy, there has been an increase in the number of people living with dementia and in people with cognitive decline. The main symptom of dementia is memory loss; it is a progressive disease that results in people becoming more impaired over time. Decline in cognitive functions, such as attention and concentration, also occurs in older people, including those who do not develop dementia. Physical activity has been identified as a protective factor in studies that examined risk factors for dementia. For people who have already developed the disease, physical activity can help to delay further decline in functioning. Studies show that there is approximately a 20% to 30% lower risk of depression and dementia for adults participating in daily physical activity. Physical activity also seems to reduce the likelihood of experiencing cognitive decline in people who do not have dementia.[29]

Impact on depression and anxiety

Physical activity can be an alternative treatment for depression. It can be used as a standalone treatment or in combination with medication and/or psychological therapy. It has few side effects and does not have the stigma that some people perceive to be attached to taking antidepressants or attending psychotherapy and counselling.

Physical activity can reduce levels of anxiety in people with mild symptoms and may also be helpful for treating clinical anxiety. Physical activity is available to all, has few costs attached, and is an empowering approach that can support self-management.

For more details about how physical activity can help increase wellbeing and prevent or manage mental health problems.

How much physical activity should I be doing?

We know all too well that that many people in the UK do not meet the current physical activity guidelines.

With an average of only 65.5% of men and 54% of women meeting the recommended physical activity levels in 2015, it is important that more people are given the knowledge and support they need to make physical activity a healthy yet enjoyable part of life.

The Department of Health recommends that adults should aim to be active daily and complete 2.5 hours of moderate intensity activity over a week – the equivalent of 30 minutes five times a week. It may sound like a lot, but it isn't as daunting as it first appears, and we have lots of suggestions to help you get started.

Where do I start?

Once you have decided that you want to be more physically active, there are a few points worth thinking about. Apart from improving your physical and mental wellbeing, what else do you want to get out of being active?

Ask yourself whether you'd prefer being indoors or out, doing a group or individual activity, or trying a new sport. If you're put off by sporty exercises, or feel uninspired at the thought of limiting yourself to just one activity, think outside the box and remember that going on a walk, doing housework, and gardening are all physical activities. Also, would you rather go it alone or do an activity with a friend? Social support is a great motivator, and sharing your experiences, goals and achievements will help you to keep focus and enthusiasm.

Overcoming barriers

It can be a bit scary making changes to your life, and most people get anxious about trying something new. Some common barriers, such as cost, injury or illness, lack of energy, fear of failure, or even the weather can hinder people from getting started; however, practical and emotional support from friends, family and experts really does help.

Body image can act as a barrier to participating in physical activity. People who are anxious about how their body will look to others while they are exercising may avoid exercise as a result. For women, attending a female-only exercise class or a ladies-only swimming session may help to overcome anxiety as a barrier to initially starting to exercise.

Exercising with a companion can also help to reduce anxiety about how your body looks to others, and may be particularly helpful during the first few exercise sessions. The environment can also influence how you feel; gyms with mirrored walls tend to heighten anxiety, as does exercising near a window or other space where you might feel 'on show'.

Make time

What time do you have available for exercise? You may need to rejig commitments to make room for extra activities, or choose something that fits into your busy schedule.

Be practical

Will you need support from friends and family to complete your chosen activities, or is there a chance your active lifestyle will have an impact on others in your life? Find out how much it will cost and, if necessary, what you can do to make it affordable.

Right for you

What kind of activity would suit you best? Think about what parts of your body you want to exercise and whether you'd prefer to be active at home or whether you fancy a change of scenery and would prefer to exercise in a different environment, indoors or outdoors.

Making it part of daily life

Adopting a more active lifestyle can be as simple as doing daily tasks more energetically or making small changes to your routine, such as walking up a flight of stairs.

Start slowly

If physical activity is new to you, it's best to build up your ability gradually. Focus on task goals, such as improving sport skills or stamina, rather than competition, and keep a record of your activity and review it to provide feedback on your progress. There are many apps and social networks accessible for free to help.

Goals

It's really important to set goals to measure progress, which might motivate you. Try using a pedometer or an app on your smartphone to measure your speed and distance travelled, or add on an extra stomach crunch or swim an extra length at the end of your session.

Remember, you won't see improvement from physical conditioning every day. Making the regular commitment to doing physical activity is an achievement in itself, and every activity session can improve your mood.

At home

There are lots of activities you can do without leaving your front door and that involve minimal cost. It can be as simple as pushing the mower with extra vigour, speeding up the housework, or doing an exercise DVD in the living room.

At work

Whether you're on your feet, sat at a desk or sat behind the wheel during your working hours, there are many ways you can get more active. Try using the stairs for journeys fewer than four floors, walking or cycling a slightly longer route home, or using your lunch hour to take a brisk walk, do an exercise class or go for a swim. The change of scenery will do you good, too.

Out and about

Being out of doors is a prime time for boosting your activity levels, and research suggests that doing physical activity in an outdoor, 'green' environment has greater positive effects on wellbeing compared to physical activity indoors.

Making small changes, from leaving the car at home for short journeys or getting off the bus a stop earlier, to higher-intensity activities like joining in with your children's football game or jogging with the dog, can help to boost your mood.

DIET AND MENTAL HEALTH

The relationship between our diet and our mental health is complex. However, research shows a link between what we eat and how we feel.

Eating well can help you feel better. You don't have to make big changes to your diet, but see if you can try some of these tips.

☐ Eat regularly. This can stop your blood sugar level dropping, which can make you feel tired and bad-tempered.

☐ Stay hydrated. Even mild dehydration can affect your mood, energy level and ability to concentrate.

☐ Eat the right balance of fats. Your brain needs healthy fats to keep working well. They're found in things such as olive oil, rapeseed oil, nuts, seeds, oily fish, avocados, milk and eggs. Avoid trans fats - often found in processed or packaged foods - as they can be bad for your mood and your heart health.

☐ Include more wholegrains, fruits and vegetables in your diet. They contain the vitamins and minerals your brain and body need to stay well.

☐ Include some protein with every meal. It contains an amino acid that your brain uses to help regulate your mood.

☐ Look after your gut health. Your gut can reflect how you're feeling: if you're stressed, it can speed up or slow down. Healthy food for your gut includes fruit, vegetables, beans and probiotics.

☐ Be aware of how caffeine can affect your mood. It can cause sleep problems, especially if you drink it close to bedtime, and some people find it makes them irritable and anxious too. Caffeine is found in coffee, tea, cola, energy drinks and chocolate.

Eating Well for Mental Health

From a young age, we're taught that eating well helps us look and feel our physical best. What we're not always told is that good nutrition significantly affects our mental health, too. A healthy, well-balanced diet can help us think clearly and feel more alert. It can also improve concentration and attention span.

Conversely, an inadequate diet can lead to fatigue, impaired decision-making, and can slow down reaction time. In fact, a poor diet can actually aggravate, and may even lead to, stress and depression.

One of the biggest health impairments is society's reliance on processed foods. These foods are high in flours and sugar and train the brain to crave more of them, rather than nutrient-rich foods such as fruits and vegetables.

A lot of the processed foods we eat are highly addictive and stimulate the dopamine centers in our brain, which are associated with pleasure and reward. In order to stop craving unhealthy foods, you've got to stop eating those foods. You actually start to change the physiology in the brain when you pull added sugars and refined carbohydrates from your diet.

Stress and Depression

Sugar and processed foods can lead to inflammation throughout the body and brain, which may contribute to mood disorders, including anxiety and depression. When we're feeling stressed or depressed, it's often processed foods we reach for in search of a quick pick-me-up. During busy or difficult periods, a cup of coffee stands in for a complete breakfast and fresh fruits and vegetables are replaced with high-fat, high-calorie fast food. When feeling down, a pint of ice cream becomes dinner (or you skip dinner altogether).

According to the American Dietetic Association, people tend to either eat too much or too little when depressed or under stress. Eat too much and you find yourself dealing with sluggishness and weight gain. Eat too little and the resulting exhaustion makes this a hard habit to break. In either case, poor diet during periods of stress and depression only makes matters worse. This cycle is a vicious one, but it can be overcome.

To boost your mental health, focus on eating plenty of fruits and vegetables along with foods rich in omega-3 fatty acids, such as salmon. Dark green leafy vegetables in particular are brain protective. Nuts, seeds and legumes, such as beans and lentils, are also excellent brain foods.

A Healthy Gut

Researchers continue to prove the old adage that you are what you eat, most recently by exploring the strong connection between our intestines and brain. Our guts and brain are physically linked via the vagus nerve, and the two are able to send messages to one another. While the gut is able to influence emotional behavior in the brain, the brain can also alter the type of bacteria living in the gut.

According to the American Psychological Association, gut bacteria produce an array of neurochemicals that the brain uses for the regulation of physiological and mental processes, including mood. It's believed 95 percent of the body's supply of serotonin, a mood stabilizer, is produced by gut bacteria.

Stress is thought to suppress beneficial gut bacteria.

Mindful Eating

Paying attention to how you feel when you eat, and what you eat, is one of the first steps in making sure you're getting well-balanced meals and snacks. Since many of us don't pay close attention to our eating habits, nutritionists recommend keeping a food journal. Documenting what, where and when you eat is a great way to gain insight into your patterns.

If you find you overeat when stressed, it may be helpful to stop what you're doing when the urge to eat arises, and to write down your feelings. By doing this, you may discover what's really bothering you. If you undereat, it may help to schedule five or six smaller meals instead of three large ones.

Sometimes, stress and depression are severe and can't be managed alone. For some, eating disorders develop. If you find it hard to control your eating habits, whether you're eating too much or too little, your health may be in jeopardy. If this is the case, you should seek professional counseling. Asking for help is never a sign of weakness or failure, especially in situations too difficult to handle alone.

Brain Food

Your brain and nervous system depend on nutrition to build new proteins, cells and tissues. In order to function effectively, your body requires a variety of carbohydrates, proteins and minerals. To get all the nutrients that improve mental functioning, nutritionists suggest eating meals and snacks that include a variety of foods, instead of eating the same meals each day.

Here are the top three foods to incorporate into a healthy mental diet:

o Complex carbohydrates — such as brown rice and starchy vegetables can give you energy. Quinoa, millet, beets and sweet potatoes have more nutritional value and will keep you satisfied longer than the simple carbohydrates found in sugar and candy.

o Lean proteins — also lend energy that allows your body to think and react quickly. Good sources of protein include chicken, meat, fish, eggs, soybeans, nuts and seeds.

o Fatty acids — are crucial for the proper function of your brain and nervous system. You can find them in fish, meat, eggs, nuts and flaxseeds.

Healthy Eating Tips

o Steer clear of processed snack foods, such as potato chips, which can impair your ability to concentrate. Pass up sugar-filled snacks, such as candy and soft drinks, which lead to ups and downs in energy levels.

o Consume plenty of healthy fats, such as olive oil, coconut oil and avocado. This will support your brain function.

o Have a healthy snack when hunger strikes, such as fruit, nuts, hard-boiled eggs, baked sweet potatoes or edamame. This will give you more energy than packaged products.

o Develop a healthy shopping list and stick to it.

o Don’t shop while hungry, since you’ll be more apt to make unhealthy impulse purchases.

o Think about where and when you eat. Don't eat in front of the television, which can be distracting and cause you to overeat. Instead, find a place to sit, relax and really notice what you're eating. Chew slowly. Savor the taste and texture.

Sharing meals with other people

There are many psychological, social and biological benefits of eating meals with other people. They give us a sense of rhythm and regularity in our lives, a chance to reflect on the day, and feel connected to others. Biologically, eating in upright chairs helps with our digestion. Talking and listening also slows us down so we don't eat too fast.

Make the most of mealtimes by setting aside at least one day a week to eat with family and friends. Choose a meal that's easy to prepare so it doesn't become a chore. Share responsibility so everyone has a different task: doing the shopping, setting the table, cooking or washing up, for example. Keep the television off so you can all talk and share.

MYTHS AND FACTS ABOUT MENTAL HEALTH

Mental Health Problems Affect Everyone

Myth: Mental health problems don't affect me.

Fact: Mental health problems are actually very common. In 2020, about:

- One in five American adults experienced a mental health issue
- One in 6 young people experienced a major depressive episode
- One in 20 Americans lived with a serious mental illness, such as schizophrenia, bipolar disorder, or major depression

Suicide is a leading cause of death in the United States. In fact, it was the 2nd leading cause of death for people ages 10-24. It accounted for the loss of more than 45,979 American lives in 2020, nearly double the number of lives lost to homicide.

Myth: Children don't experience mental health problems.

Fact: Even very young children may show early warning signs of mental health concerns. These mental health problems are often clinically diagnosable, and can be a product of the interaction of biological, psychological, and social factors.

Half of all mental health disorders show first signs before a person turns 14 years old, and three-quarters of mental health disorders begin before age 24.

Unfortunately, only half of children and adolescents with diagnosable mental health problems receive the treatment they need. Early mental health support can help a child before problems interfere with other developmental needs.

Myth: People with mental health problems are violent and unpredictable.

Fact: The vast majority of people with mental health problems are no more likely to be violent than anyone else. Most people with mental illness are not violent and only 3%–5% of violent acts can be attributed to individuals living with a serious mental illness. In fact, people with severe mental illnesses are over 10 times more likely to be victims of violent crime than the general population. You probably know someone with a mental health problem and don't even realize it, because many people with mental health problems are highly active and productive members of our communities.

Myth: People with mental health needs, even those who are managing their mental illness, cannot tolerate the stress of holding down a job.

Fact: People with mental health problems are just as productive as other employees. Employers who hire people with mental health problems report good attendance and punctuality as well as motivation, good work, and job tenure on par with or greater than other employees.

When employees with mental health problems receive effective treatment, it can result in:

- Lower total medical costs
- Increased productivity
- Lower absenteeism
- Decreased disability costs

Myth: Personality weakness or character flaws cause mental health problems. People with mental health problems can snap out of it if they try hard enough.

Fact: Mental health problems have nothing to do with being lazy or weak and many people need help to get better. Many factors contribute to mental health problems, including:

- Biological factors, such as genes, physical illness, injury, or brain chemistry
- Life experiences, such as trauma or a history of abuse
- Family history of mental health problems

People with mental health problems can get better and many recover completely.

Helping Individuals with Mental Health Problems

Myth: There is no hope for people with mental health problems. Once a friend or family member develops mental health problems, he or she will never recover.

Fact: Studies show that people with mental health problems get better and many recover completely. Recovery refers to the process in which people are able to live, work, learn, and participate fully in their communities. There are more treatments, services, and community support systems than ever before, and they work.

Myth: Therapy and self-help are a waste of time. Why bother when you can just take a pill?

Fact: Treatment for mental health problems varies depending on the individual and could include medication, therapy, or both. Many individuals work with a support system during the healing and recovery process.

Myth: I can't do anything for a person with a mental health problem.

Fact: Friends and loved ones can make a big difference. In 2020, only 20% of adults received any mental health treatment in the past year, which included 10% who received counseling or therapy from a professional. Friends and family can be important influences to help someone get the treatment and services they need by:

- Reaching out and letting them know you are available to help
- Helping them access mental health services
- Learning and sharing the facts about mental health, especially if you hear something that isn't true
- Treating them with respect, just as you would anyone else

- Refusing to define them by their diagnosis or using labels such as "crazy", instead use person-first language

Myth: Prevention doesn't work. It is impossible to prevent mental illnesses.

Fact: Prevention of mental, emotional, and behavioral disorders focuses on addressing known risk factors such as exposure to trauma that can affect the chances that children, youth, and young adults will develop mental health problems. Promoting the social-emotional well-being of children and youth leads to:

- Higher overall productivity
- Better educational outcomes

- Lower crime rates
- Stronger economies
- Lower health care costs
- Improved quality of life
- Increased lifespan
- Improved family life

CONCLUSION

It is absolutely vital to speak up when you're struggling and seek professional guidance for assistance in managing your symptoms if you have a mood disorder. Since mood disorders look different for every individual, your treatment plan should be tailored to your specific needs and situation.

While mood disorders can be episodic, they can also present a lifelong vulnerability. Treatment should be focused on the management of symptoms to minimize their impact on your daily life.

Most importantly, keep in mind that a mood disorder in no way defines you or dictates how full of a life you can lead. Many people with mood disorders lead happy and fulfilling lives by managing their symptoms through a combination of therapy, medication, and self-care.

www.ingramcontent.com/pod-product-compliance
Lightning Source LLC
LaVergne TN
LVHW050316160826
845677LV00014B/3420

* 9 7 9 8 3 7 0 4 4 9 0 8 6 *